The Complete Cleansing Guide for Beginners

How to Lose Weight Fast to Optimize Your Health, Revitalize Your Appearance & Rapidly Increase Your Energy Through Cleanse Diets

Melanie Wyatt

Table Of Contents

Introduction

I want to thank you and congratulate you for purchasing the book, "**Cleansing Guide for Beginners**: *How to Lose Weight Fast to Optimize Your Health, Revitalize Your Appearance & Rapidly Increase Your Energy Through Cleanse Diets.*"

This book contains proven steps and strategies on how to effectively undertake a cleansing diet program to lose weight fast and optimize your overall health.

This book also provides some sample cleansing diet recipes and tips to boost your weight loss and boost your energy level.

Thanks again for purchasing this book, I hope you enjoy it! Please take some time to stop by and LIKE our Facebook page:

https://www.facebook.com/joypublishing

With gratitude,

Melanie Wyatt

Chapter 1 - Cleanse Basics: What You Need to Know about Cleanse Diet

Cleanse diet has become a very popular way to get healthy and lose excess weight. It is important to know how to do the cleanse diet properly in order to feel good and stay healthy.

The cleanse diet is actually not a new thing. In the United States, cleanse diet became popular in the 1920s and 1930s. However, when the theories backing it lost support, it slowly fell out of favor. Currently, the idea of cleansing with the use of colon irrigation, enzymes or teas has experienced resurgence.

What is Cleanse?

The definition of cleanse is quite extensive. In its basic sense, cleanse is any type of lifestyle regimen or diet which is focused at detoxifying the body and bringing back optimum health. The sad part is, cleanse or cleansing is usually synonymous with eating disordered. However, cleansing can possibly be a vital part of a weight loss regimen if you use the right kind of cleanse or detox diet appropriate for your body and lifestyle.

What is the theory behind natural cleanse?

One of the primary theories behind cleanse or cleansing is a traditional belief referred to as the theory of autointoxication. The principle behind this belief is that the undigested food may lead to the buildup of mucus in the colon. This accumulation generates toxins, which poisons the body as it enters the bloodstream.

Most people reported that these toxins can lead to different symptoms, including the following:

- Low energy

- Weight gain

- Headache

- Fatigue

What is natural cleanse?

There are two primary methods of cleanse or cleansing: One involves seeing a health practitioner to have colon irrigation; and the other involves buying and using cleansing products.

1. Cleansing with colon irrigation (high colonics). Colonic hydrotherapists or colonic hygienists conduct colon irrigations. Colon irrigations work like an enema, although they involve no discomfort and odors and much more water. During colon irrigation, you lie on a table, and then a gravity-based reservoir or a low-pressure pump flushes several gallons of water through a tiny tube that's inserted into the rectum.

   A therapist may massage the abdomen after the water is in the colon. The water is then released like a regular bowel movement. This procedure flushes out the wastes and fluids. The whole process may be repeated. A session may usually last up to an hour.

   The health care provider may use various temperatures and water pressures. The use of probiotics, coffee, herbs and enzymes may also be employed.

2. Cleansing with the use of liquid or powdered supplements. This involves taking some supplements for cleansing by mouth or taken through the rectum. Either way, the principle behind this is to help the colon get rid of its contents. These cleansing products may be bought in supermarkets, pharmacies or health food stores. They include:

- Magnesium

- Enzymes

- Herbal teas

- Laxatives – both stimulant and non-stimulant kinds

- Enemas

What is the Goal of Cleansing?

Colon irrigation practitioners and producers of colon cleansing products claim broad and wide-reaching health benefits of cleansing. Their ultimate objective is to clean up the colon from huge amounts of stagnant, potentially toxic waste accumulated on the colon walls. Doing a cleanse, as they claim, will improve the natural vigor of the body.

Other stated goals of doing a cleanse include the following:

- Lessening the risk of developing colon cancer

- Weight loss

- Boosting the immune system

- Improving mental outlook

Cleansing has been the subject of studies in relation to a number of health issues, including the following:

- Before and during bowel surgeries

- Drug withdrawal

- Spasm during colonoscopy

- Ostomy or the surgical relation between the outside of the body and the intestine

- Fecal incontinence

Chapter 2: The Benefits of a Cleanse Diet

Cleansing diets can help in improving the body's general health and wellness. It can even reduce the risks of developing colon cancer. Below is a list of some of the claimed benefits of a cleanse diet:

1. Enhances the body's well-being. Cleansing the colon from toxins and wastes may be achieved by releasing layers of colon buildup. This can bring about feelings of strength and lightness, as well as overall good health and well being.

2. Maintains proper pH balance in the bloodstream. Foods that lead to colon blockages produce acids, specifically diet abundant in protein without sufficient fiber. This results to overall malaise in the body. The tissues in the colon eventually become inflamed and damaged, weakening the colon. The colon may not be effective in its function of allowing only vitamins, minerals and water to pass into the bloodstream. If fecal matter, parasites, fungus, molds and yeasts enter the bloodstream and connected tissue, the pH level of the body will be thrown out of balance.

3. Enhances fertility. Cleanse diet involves the intake of increased amounts of fiber and health food choices. It also keeps weight under control. Fat is based on estrogen. If too

much fat is present, the chance of becoming pregnant is relatively low. A colon which is weighed down by years of accumulation can also adversely affect the uterus, as well as the surrounding reproductive organs in females, causing strain.

Cleansing diet helps in ridding the body of many toxins and harmful chemicals that adversely affect the sperm and egg. A lot of natural health practitioners suggest that both partners try cleansing diets before attempting pregnancy.

4. Lessens the risk of developing colon cancer. All the toxic substances that you breathe in, drink, eat and absorb through the skin are broken down by the liver and gastrointestinal system. If these harmful substances are not eliminated from the liver and colon as fast as possible, they can damage the body's systems. By getting rid of stagnant body waste, you lessen the causes and risk of developing cancerous growths, cysts and polyps in the colon and the gastrointestinal tract.

5. Kick-starts weight loss. Food items, which are low in fiber, transport through the digestive tract at a much slower pace than those that are abundant in fiber. These slow-moving food items generate excess mucous that tend to stick to the walls of the intestine. This will eventually drag down the intestinal tract with excess pounds of decaying fecal materials.

Cleansing diet also helps in weight reduction. Many people have claimed to lose weight up to 20 pounds over only a month. A cleansing diet can lead to dramatic weight loss and jump-start your metabolism. It can also lead your interests to better food choices and overall wellness.

6. Enhances concentration. Ineffective vitamin absorption as well as poor diet can make you more distracted and lose concentration. The accumulation of mucous and toxic substances in the colon can prevent the body from obtaining what it needs to function optimally. Cleaning up the colon with a cleansing diet can be the key to better concentration and alertness. Its effects can greatly affect your overall health, and also your work and relationships.

7. Boosts the body's ability to effectively absorb vitamins and nutrients. A clean colon works effectively in allowing only vitamins, nutrients and water to be absorbed into the bloodstream, rather than releasing bacteria and toxic material through the walls of the colon. When the colon is cleansed, it clears up the way for important vitamins and nutrients to filter into the body unhampered

8. Enhances the digestive system's effectiveness. As the colon is cleansed, it eliminates undigested wastes out of the body, clearing the way for the good nutrients to be absorbed effectively. If the toxic materials and wastes stay in the body for a long time, it becomes a breeding ground for illnesses and bad bacteria. A clean colon through a

cleansing diet allows toxic materials from undigested waste to pass easily through the digestive tract.

9. Maintains the regularity of bowel movements and prevents constipation. Constipation, particularly when it is chronic, leads to sluggish digestive response. This will make the wastes stay longer in the digestive system. This condition will increase the chances of toxic materials released into the bloodstream. This will become the cause of irritations and other health problems such as varicose veins and hemorrhoids.

Chapter 3: Top 14 Cleansing Foods

Food is really the best form of medicine when it comes to cleansing the body of harmful toxins. You will be amazed to find out that a lot of your favorite foods can cleanse the body's natural detoxification organs such as the skin, kidneys, intestines and liver. Cleansing will prevent harmful toxic accumulation. Help in ridding the adverse effects of second-hand smoke, food additives, pollution and other toxins by eating healthy and delicious foods such as the following:

1. Cabbage – contains a number of antioxidant and anticancer substances that help the liver in breaking down excessive hormones. Cabbage can also cleanse the digestive tract and maintain some of the harmful substances found in cigarette fumes at bay. Cabbage can also boost the liver's natural ability to detoxify.

2. Blueberries – is one of the most potent healing foods. Blueberries have natural aspirin that aids in reducing the tissue-damaging impacts of chronic inflammation, while reducing pain. It also serves as antibiotics by hampering bacterial entry in the urinary tract, thereby assisting in the prevention of infection. Blueberries also contain antiviral components which help in blocking toxins from crossing blood-brain barrier to obtain access to the delicate brain.

3. Beets – contain a peculiar combination of natural plant substances which make them effective liver cleansers and blood purifiers.

4. Avocados – are nutritional powerhouses that can dilate blood vessels and lessen cholesterol levels while blocking artery-damaging toxicity. Avocados contain a natural compound called glutathione, which blocks at least 30 various carcinogenic substances while helping the liver's natural ability to detoxify synthetic substances.

5. Apples – are abundant in pectin, which is a kind of fiber that binds heavy metals and cholesterol in the body. Apples help largely in getting rid of toxin accumulation and cleansing the colon.

6. Grapefruit – contains an abundant amount of pectin, which is a type of fiber that binds cholesterol molecules in the body, thereby cleansing the blood. Pectin fiber also binds heavy metals in the body as they are flushed out of the digestive system. Grapefruit also contains antiviral substances which help in cleansing dangerous viruses out of the body. Grapefruit is a potent liver and intestinal detoxifier.

7. Garlic – helps in cleansing viruses, intestinal parasites and harmful bacteria from the body, particularly in the intestines and the blood. Garlic also aids in cleansing build up in the arteries and contain antioxidant and anti-cancer

properties that help detoxify the body of dangerous substances. In addition to this, it helps with the cleansing of the respiratory tract by getting rid of mucus accumulation in the sinuses and the lungs. Choose only fresh garlic to take advantage of its numerous health benefits and not powdered garlic, which virtually does not contain any of the above-mentioned properties.

8. Flaxseeds and flaxseed oil – contain abundant levels of essential fatty acids, specifically Omega 3. Flaxseed oil and flaxseed are important for a lot of cleansing activities all throughout the body.

9. Celery and celery seed – are potent blood cleansers. They also contain a variety of anti-cancer substances that aid in detoxifying cancer cells out of the body. Celery and celery seeds have over twenty different anti-inflammatory compounds which are specifically excellent for cleansing compounds found in cigarette fumes.

10. Watercress – this delicious green may not be familiar for many but this can be an excellent choice for sandwiches since it can boost the activity of detoxification enzymes and acts on any present cancer cells throughout the body. According to current clinical studies, watercress can eliminate higher than average amounts of carcinogenic compounds among smokers, thereby eliminating them from the body.

11. Seaweed – while seaweed may have been the most underrated vegetable in western communities, according to scientific research, seaweeds bind to heavy metal waste in the body. Seaweed can also bind to radioactive wastes inside the body to help in flushing them out. Furthermore, seaweed is a powerhouse of trace minerals.

12. Lemons – contain huge amounts of Vitamin C, which makes them excellent liver detoxifiers. Vitamin C is required by the body to make an essential compound called glutathione, which aids the liver in detoxifying dangerous compounds in the body. To support your cleansing efforts regularly, add a squeeze of fresh lemon juice to pure water.

13. Legumes – are abundant with fiber that aids in reducing cholesterol levels, regulates blood sugar levels and cleanses the intestines. They also aid in safeguarding the body against all types of cancer.

14. Kale – contains potent antioxidant and anti-cancer properties that aid in cleansing the body of dangerous compounds. Kale is also abundant in fiber, which assists in cleansing the intestinal tract. Just as like cabbage, kelp aids balance out the compounds found in cigarette fumes and boosts the natural ability of the liver for cleansing.

Chapter 4 Some Popular Types of Cleansing Diet Plans

A cleansing diet is also commonly referred to as "detox diet". A cleansing diet helps in getting rid of harmful toxins and poisons out of the body. The basic principle of an effective and powerful cleansing diet program is to eat fresh and organic food items, which will promote the effective functioning of the kidneys, liver and the lymphatic system. Below are some of the most popular kinds of a cleansing diet

Raw Food Cleansing Diet

1. Raw Food Cleansing Diet — Involves a dietary plan which basically introduces the beneficial effects of raw foods. This diet plan also includes a wide range of cleansing selections which lasts from 3 to 28 days.

2. Raw Food Detox Diet Plan — A meal plan which involves the slow incorporation of raw foods into the everyday diet to promote detoxification

3. The Remedy — A diet program which is based on raw foods as well as green juices.

This diet plan involves a 5-week program which provides for a slow adjustment period from a normal eating habit to a raw vegan diet

4.	28 Day Raw Detox	A dietary plan which is based on raw vegan diet in conjunction with various choices of whole food nutritional supplements
5.	Quantum Eating	A meal plan which is based on raw foods that can detoxify the body and promotes youthfulness
6.	Hallelujah Diet	A meal plan designed by George Malkus. This diet program is bible-based.

Popular Cleansing Diet Meal Plans

1.	The Master Cleanse Diet / Lemon Diet	This cleansing diet program is considered to be the most popular, short-term cleansing program because of its large media coverage.
2.	Beauty Detox Solution	This meal plan is intended for people who are interested in a gentle process that is sustainable

for a long term lifestyle. The Beauty Detox Solution diet program presents an approach to a healthier eating habit which aids in cleansing the body and promote the overall health and beauty.

3.	Sugar Detox	This diet plan lasts for 31 days. It helps in getting rid of sugar addiction while you start taking the path towards having a healthier eating habit. This diet program particularly helps a person control the blood sugar levels to improve skin tone, gets rid of unwanted weight and improves energy levels.
4.	Easy Body Cleansing Diets	This diet program provides various cleansing diet plans which are intended to reap the benefits of different health goals and conditions.
5.	The Clean Diet	This meal program lasts for 21 days. It is widely popularized by Dr. Alejandro Junger and is particularly intended for people who have a busy lifestyle.

6. Clean Green and Lean	This diet program lasts for 4 weeks which helps a person to overcome chronic health issues including fatigue.
7. Clean Gut	This diet plan is intended to cleanse the intestines to address different kinds of health issues and illnesses.
8. Detox Diet for Women	This diet program is particularly intended for females. It promotes cleansing but in a way that is less invasive on the dieter's lifestyle.
9. Detox Prescription	A diet plan which provides various cleansing selections to suit any types of lifestyle
10. Detox Strategy	This meal plan provides an in-depth information on toxins and outlines a comprehensive lifestyle plan. The Detox Strategy program is backed up by principles based on clinical researches to cleanse and detoxify the body.

11. Diuretic Diet The diet program which reduces fluid retention through the use of natural diuretics.

12. Eating for Energy: Living Foods Diet This diet program allows the dieters to slowly change their eating patterns by providing a flexible approach. This program provides special information that specifically applies to physically active dieters as well as athletes. This diet plan is based on a detox component in conjunction with a diet program.

13. Eat Stop Eat This diet plan enhances detox by using short-24 hour fasts during a couple of times every week.

14. Mucusless Diet This diet program is designed by Arnold Ehret in his book entitled "Mucusless Diet Healing System". This diet program is said to have cured Arnold Ehret from Bright's disease.

15. Lose Weight without Working out or Dieting — This diet meal plan provides long-term weight loss by cleansing the body with the use of slimming nutrient-based foods.

Chapter 5 Cleansing Diet Sample Recipes and Tips

SNACKS

Chips made of Kale

Ingredients

- 2 tbsp nutritional yeast

- A bunch of kale (about 6 ounces)

- 1 tbsp olive oil

- Sea salt to taste

Procedure:

1. Pre-heat the oven at 300 degrees Fahrenheit.

2. Rinse and thoroughly dry the kale. Cut the stems and the tough core ribs and cut into big pieces.

3. In a large bowl, toss in the kale with olive oil.

23

4. Sprinkle with sea salt to taste.

5. In a big baking sheet, arrange the kale leaves in one layer.

6. Bake until crisp or about 20 minutes.

7. In a rack, cool the baking sheet and serve.

Roasted Chickpeas

Ingredients

- A combination of your favorite spices such as, dill and nutritional yeast, thyme or paprika and nutritional yeast or sea salt

- A whole can of chickpeas

Procedure:

1. Open the can of chickpeas and dry the contents with towel paper.

2. Place the towel-dried chickpeas in a large baking sheet.

3. Bake in the oven for 400 degrees Fahrenheit. Roast until crisp and brown or about 30 minutes.

4. In a large bowl, combine all the ingredients and then toss in the hot chickpeas. Serve while warm.

DRINKS

Spa Water with Cucumber, Mint and Lime

Ingredients:

- Cucumber slices

- Lime Juice

- Fresh Mint

- Filtered Water

Procedure:

1. In a large ceramic or glass pitcher, put the ingredients all together.

2. Keep the mixture and store in the chiller for at least a couple of hours.

3. The mixture can be drink within a few days.

Clean Lemonade

Ingredients:

- Stevia (to taste)

- 2 medium sized lemons, juiced

- 8 ounces of filtered water or soda water

Procedure:

1. Mix in the ingredients all together.

2. Store in the refrigerator and enjoy within a few days

Cleansing Hot Chocolate

Ingredients

- Raw cacao (to taste)

- Stevia (to taste)

- Cinnamon or mint extract (optional)

- Almond or coconut milk

Procedure:

1. Warm the milk on a stove top.

2. Add the chocolate according to taste.

3. Serve while warm

Additional Tips When Undertaking a Cleansing Diet Program

When undertaking a cleansing program, the liver will require more nutrients. In addition to this, increasing the flow of bile is also considered as a crucial part of an effective cleansing program. This is because the bile is responsible for transporting fat-soluble toxic materials away from the liver which is eliminated out of the body through bowels. Some of the signs of poor flow of bile include the following:

- Indigestion after consuming fat-rich foods

- Dry skin and hair

- Indigestion after 1-2 hours after eating

- Flatulence

- Constipation

- Small hard stools

When undergoing a cleansing program, you will need enough supply of the following essential vitamins and nutrients to make your detox program more effective:

1. Vitamin C – a water soluble vitamin which contains anti-oxidative components that support the process of cleansing. This essential vitamin also aids in reducing a number of different cleansing side effects including headache and nausea.

2. Multivitamins – when undertaking a cleansing program, select a high-potency multivitamin that contains enough dosage of selenium, molybdenum and zinc, among others.

3. Choline and Methionine – these nutrients are also known as lipotropic factors, which aid in the regulation of fat metabolism and increasing bile flow.

4. Protein – is required in sufficient amounts by the liver for an effective cleansing process. Protein may be obtained from sources such as beans, quinoa, protein powder and nuts. There are a few people who may opt to eat exclusively fish but only in moderation.

Conclusion

Thank you again for purchasing this book!

I hope this book was able to help you to have a comprehensive understanding about cleansing diets and its numerous benefits.

The next step is to try out some of the cleansing diet recipes and tips and say hello to a leaner and healthier you.

Finally, please remember to check out our Facebook page in order to find other resources and upcoming promotions:

https://www.facebook.com/joypublishing

With sincere thanks,

Melanie Wyatt

One Last Thing...

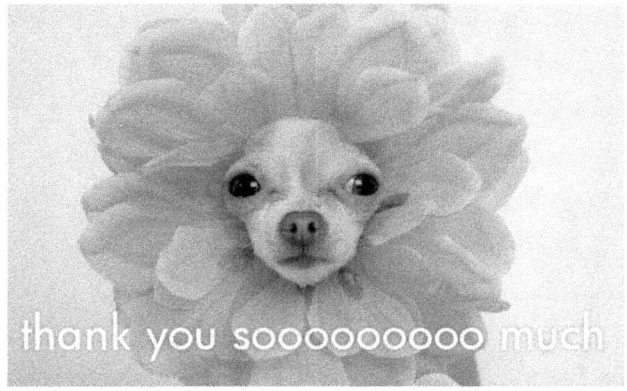

If you believe that this book is worth sharing, would you please take the time to let others know how it affected your life? If it turns out to make a difference in the lives of others, they will be forever grateful to you, as will I.

www.ingramcontent.com/pod-product-compliance
Lightning Source LLC
Chambersburg PA
CBHW070517290526
45790CB00003B/1251